2023 OPTIMAL PRENATAL NUTRITION

Prenatal omega-3 sources

Prossy press

Copyright 2023

Table of Contents

- *Folic acid*
- *Iron supplements*
- *Vitamin*
- *Fortification*

Conclusion

Introduction

Prenatal nutrition is a vital aspect in the health and development of both the mother and her developing baby. Optimal nutrition throughout pregnancy is vital for maintaining healthy growth and development of the fetus, minimizing the risk of pregnancy problems, and enhancing the long-term health of both the mother and the infant. The dietary choices a woman makes during pregnancy may have a tremendous influence on the health of her developing baby, and it is crucial for women to be attentive of their nutritional requirements during this critical time.

The first trimester of pregnancy is a key stage for the growth of the baby. During this stage, the baby's brain, heart, and other essential organs begin to develop. Adequate consumption of critical nutrients such as folic acid, iron, and calcium is needed to promote this growth and development. Folic acid, in particular, is necessary for the creation of the neural tube, which ultimately becomes the brain and spinal cord. Iron is vital to maintain the developing baby's increasing blood volume, while calcium is needed for healthy bones and teeth.

In the second and third trimesters, the fetus continues to grow and develop at a fast speed, and the mother's nutritional demands also rise. Protein is required for the development and repair of tissues, and it is crucial for the mother to consume enough quantities of high-quality protein sources such as lean meats, poultry, fish, beans, and dairy products. In addition, the baby's increased need for iron may lead to iron-deficiency anemia in the mother if she does not take appropriate iron from dietary sources such as red meat, chicken, and iron-fortified cereals.

It is also vital for women to restrict their use of certain foods and drugs during pregnancy. Caffeine, for example, should be minimized, since it might pass the placenta and influence the baby's heart rate and sleep habits. Alcohol should be avoided altogether, since it may damage the growing baby and raise the chance of birth abnormalities and behavioral issues. Women should also avoid raw or undercooked meat, seafood with high mercury levels, and unpasteurized dairy products, since these meals may contain hazardous bacteria or poisons that might damage the developing baby.

In addition to concentrating on certain nutrients, women should attempt to have a balanced and diverse diet throughout pregnancy. This involves incorporating a range of fruits and vegetables, healthy grains, and lean protein sources in their meals. It is also vital for women to maintain a healthy weight and prevent excessive weight gain during pregnancy. Gaining too much weight during pregnancy may raise the risk of pregnancy disorders such as gestational diabetes and pre-eclampsia, and it can also make it more difficult to shed weight following pregnancy.

Finally, it is crucial for women to consult with their healthcare professionals to design a tailored dietary plan that suits their particular requirements and the needs of their developing baby. This may require monitoring nutritional levels, such as iron and calcium, and making modifications to their meals as appropriate. Women should also be careful of their calorie demands during pregnancy, since it is crucial to eat enough calories to support the growth and development of the baby.

In conclusion, adequate prenatal nutrition is a vital aspect in the health and development of both the mother and her developing child. Women should concentrate on having a balanced and diverse diet that contains enough levels of critical nutrients, limiting their consumption of specific foods and substances, and maintaining a healthy weight. With the supervision of their healthcare experts, women may ensure that they and their developing kids get the food they need to promote a successful pregnancy and a bright future.

Importance of Prenatal Nutrition

Prenatal nutrition is crucial for both the health of the mother and the growth of the baby. Adequate nutrition during pregnancy promotes the growth and development of the baby and helps to avoid certain health concerns in the mother. Here are some of the primary advantages of excellent prenatal nutrition:

Supports fetal growth: Proper diet throughout pregnancy helps ensure that the baby obtains the required nutrients for growth and development. This contains the building blocks for the brain and neurological system, as well as the production of organs, bones, and muscles.

Prevents birth defects: Adequate consumption of certain nutrients, such as folic acid, may help avoid birth abnormalities of the brain and spinal cord.

Increases energy levels: Pregnancy may be physically demanding, and adequate eating can help keep energy levels up. Eating a balanced diet that contains whole grains, lean protein, and healthy fats will assist sustain energy levels throughout the day.

Supports maternal health: Proper nutrition during pregnancy may help avoid health concerns in the mother, such as gestational diabetes, high blood pressure, and pre-eclampsia.

Helps prevent excessive weight gain: Pregnancy is not the time to shed weight, but it is also not the time to indulge in junk food and excessive calorie consumption. Gaining too much weight during pregnancy might raise the risk of difficulties and make it tougher to shed weight once the baby is delivered.

To promote proper prenatal nutrition, it is crucial to consume a balanced and diverse diet that contains enough fruits, vegetables, whole grains, lean protein, and healthy fats. It is also vital to avoid specific meals, such as raw or undercooked meat, seafood with high amounts of mercury, and unpasteurized dairy products.

In addition to food, vitamins may play a role in prenatal nutrition. Women who are pregnant or attempting to conceive should take a daily prenatal vitamin that includes folic acid and iron, as well as other critical vitamins and minerals.

Finally, it is crucial to keep hydrated throughout pregnancy. Drinking lots of water and avoiding sugary beverages will help keep energy levels up and prevent dehydration.

In conclusion, prenatal nutrition is vital for the health of both the mother and the baby. Eating a balanced diet, taking prenatal vitamins, and keeping hydrated will help guarantee a healthy pregnancy and the best possible result for both mother and baby.

Chapter 1: Macronutrients for optimal prenatal nutrition

A. Proteins

Proteins are one of the essential macronutrients that play a critical role in providing optimal nutrition for pregnant women. Proteins are the building blocks of the human body and are necessary for growth, repair, and maintenance of tissues, including the fetus, placenta, and uterus. They are also involved in the production of hormones, enzymes, and immune cells.

Adequate protein intake during pregnancy is crucial for proper fetal development, particularly during the second and third trimesters when the fetus experiences the most growth. During this time, the demand for protein increases to support the growth of the fetus, placenta, and uterus. It's essential that pregnant women consume enough protein to meet this increased demand.

When considering protein sources, it's important to choose those that are high in quality and bioavailability. High-quality proteins are those that contain all nine essential amino acids, which are the building blocks of proteins. Good sources of high-quality protein include meat, poultry, fish, eggs, dairy products, soy products, and legumes. These protein sources are also rich in other essential nutrients, such as iron, zinc, and B-vitamins, which are important for the health of the fetus and the mother.

It's recommended that pregnant women consume about 71 grams of protein per day, which is about 25 grams more than the recommended amount for non-pregnant women. This increased need for protein can be met through a balanced diet that includes a variety of protein-rich foods.

However, some pregnant women may have special dietary needs, such as those with gestational diabetes or vegetarian or vegan diets. For these women, it's important to consult a registered dietitian who can provide personalized nutrition recommendations.

In addition to providing essential building blocks for the fetus, protein also plays a role in the mother's health during pregnancy. It helps to maintain blood sugar levels, reduces the risk of preeclampsia, and promotes a healthy weight gain. During pregnancy, weight gain is necessary to support the growing fetus, but it's important that the weight gain is gradual and in line with the guidelines set by the healthcare provider.

Another important role of protein during pregnancy is to help the mother maintain muscle mass. As the uterus expands, the mother's abdominal muscles and back muscles may experience stress, leading to fatigue and discomfort. Consuming adequate protein can help to maintain muscle mass and reduce the risk of muscle strain.

In conclusion, proteins are an essential macronutrient for optimal prenatal nutrition. Adequate protein intake during pregnancy is necessary to support the growth of the fetus and promote a healthy pregnancy. Pregnant women should consume high-quality protein sources, such as meat, poultry, fish, eggs, dairy products, soy products, and legumes, and aim to consume about 71 grams of protein per day. Women with special dietary needs should consult a registered dietitian for personalized nutrition recommendations.

B. Fats

Fats are an important component of a balanced and nutritious diet, particularly during pregnancy. As a macronutrient, they supply the body with needed fatty acids, energy, and support many physiological activities. Pregnant women need a balanced diet of all macronutrients, including fats, to promote the growth and development of the fetus and preserve their own health.

There are three basic kinds of fats: saturated, unsaturated, and trans fats. Saturated fats, widely found in animal products, are normally solid at room temperature and may elevate cholesterol levels. Unsaturated fats, particularly monounsaturated and polyunsaturated fats, are normally liquid at room temperature and have a favorable influence on cholesterol levels. Trans fats, which are widely present in processed foods, have a harmful influence on heart health and should be avoided.

During pregnancy, it is suggested that women strive for a balanced consumption of both unsaturated and saturated fats, with a focus on unsaturated fats. This may be done by introducing a range of healthy fats into the diet, such as olive oil, avocados, almonds, and fatty seafood such as salmon and sardines.

One of the most significant unsaturated fats during pregnancy is omega-3 fatty acids. Omega-3 fatty acids are important fatty acids that the body cannot generate itself, making it vital to receive them from the food. They play a key function in the development of the fetus, including brain, eye, and nervous system development. In addition, omega-3 fatty acids have been proven to lessen the incidence of pre-eclampsia, a potentially dangerous condition during pregnancy. Fatty fish, such as salmon, sardines, and anchovies, are some of the richest sources of omega-3 fatty acids.

Another unsaturated lipid that is beneficial during pregnancy is monounsaturated fat, often found in olive oil, avocados, and almonds. This form of fat has been demonstrated to enhance blood sugar management, cut cholesterol levels, and reduce the risk of heart disease. In addition, monounsaturated fats are a wonderful source of energy and may assist to maintain a healthy weight throughout pregnancy.

It is vital to restrict the consumption of saturated and trans fats during pregnancy, since they may lead to an increased risk of heart disease and other health concerns. Saturated fats are typically found in animal products, such as meat, dairy, and butter, and should be taken in moderation. Trans fats, typically found in processed meals such as fried dishes and baked products, should be avoided totally.

In addition to delivering necessary fatty acids and energy, fats also play a role in absorbing and transporting fat-soluble vitamins such as vitamins A, D, E, and K. These vitamins are vital for the growth and development of the fetus and the health of the mother.

In conclusion, fats are a vital component of a balanced diet during pregnancy, supplying needed fatty acids, energy, and supporting many physiological activities. It is vital to strive for a balanced consumption of both unsaturated and saturated fats, with a focus on unsaturated fats, while reducing the intake of trans fats. By introducing a range of healthy fats into the diet, such as olive oil, avocados, almonds, and fatty fish, pregnant women may guarantee they are supplying their bodies and their fetuses with the vital nutrients required for optimum health and development.

C. Carbohydrates

Carbohydrates are a kind of macronutrient that plays a critical function in prenatal nutrition. They are the body's principal source of energy, supplying food for the mother's body and her developing fetus. In this post, we will investigate the advantages of carbohydrates in prenatal nutrition and how they help to a healthy pregnancy.

Carbohydrates are made up of sugar molecules, which are broken down into glucose in the body. Glucose is the body's major source of energy, and it is vital for the efficient functioning of the brain and other organs. During pregnancy, the need for glucose rises as the developing baby requires energy for its growth. To fulfill this increased need, it is vital for pregnant women to eat a balanced and enough quantity of carbs.

Carbohydrates are categorized into two types: simple and complicated. Simple carbs, also known as simple sugars, are present in meals such as candies, sweets, and fruit. Complex carbs, on the other hand, are found in meals such as whole grains, legumes, and vegetables. Simple carbs give a fast source of energy, but they are easily digested and may induce increases in blood sugar levels. On the other hand, complex carbs offer a gradual and continuous supply of energy and are a vital component of a balanced diet.

During pregnancy, the recommended daily consumption of carbohydrates is between 175 and 225 grams. This is comparable to around 45% to 65% of a pregnant woman's overall calorie consumption. Complex carbs, such as whole grains, legumes, and vegetables, should make up the bulk of a pregnant woman's carbohydrate consumption. These foods are high in fiber, which helps to manage blood sugar levels and maintain a healthy weight. Whole grains, for example, are also a rich source of B vitamins, which play a critical role in fetal growth and ensuring a healthy pregnancy.

In addition to supplying energy, carbohydrates are also needed for normal fetal growth. For example, carbohydrates are a crucial component of the placenta, which provides the growing fetus with nutrients, oxygen, and waste removal. Proper placental function is vital for the healthy growth and development of the fetus, and a lack of carbohydrates in the mother's diet can negatively impact the placenta's ability to function.

Furthermore, carbohydrates also play a crucial role in the development of the fetus's central nervous system. The brain is the largest consumer of glucose in the body, and during pregnancy, the demand for glucose in the brain increases. As a result, pregnant women need to consume a sufficient amount of carbohydrates to ensure that their growing fetus has the energy it needs to develop a healthy brain and central nervous system.

One important thing to note is that pregnant women should avoid consuming refined carbohydrates, such as white bread and sugary drinks. These types of carbohydrates are rapidly absorbed by the body, which can cause spikes in blood sugar levels and increase the risk of gestational diabetes. Instead, pregnant women should focus on consuming complex carbohydrates, such as whole grains, legumes, and vegetables, which provide a slow and sustained source of energy and are a rich source of fiber.

In conclusion, carbs constitute a vital component of prenatal nutrition. They provide energy to the mother's body and her growing fetus and are essential for proper fetal development and a healthy pregnancy. By eating a balanced and suitable quantity of carbohydrates, pregnant women may guarantee that their developing fetus gets the energy it needs for optimal growth and development. So, it is advisable for pregnant women to consume a variety of healthy carbohydrates, such as whole grains, legumes, and vegetables, and avoid consuming refined carbohydrates, such as white bread and sugary drinks.

Chapter2: Micronutrients

A. Folate

Folate, often known as vitamin B9, is a micronutrient that plays a key role in prenatal nutrition. It is an important vitamin that is crucial for the proper development of the fetus and offers several advantages for both the mother and the developing kid. In this post, we will investigate the relevance of folate in prenatal nutrition and how it contributes to a healthy pregnancy.

Folate is involved in various critical activities in the body, including DNA synthesis and cell division. During pregnancy, the requirement for folate rises as the baby is quickly expanding and dividing. As a consequence, it is necessary for pregnant women to take an adequate quantity of folate to ensure that their developing baby receives the nutrients it requires for normal growth.

Folate is present in a number of foods, including leafy green vegetables, legumes, nuts, and fruits. Pregnant women are urged to ingest at least 600 micrograms of folate each day, which may be gained via a balanced diet or with a prenatal vitamin supplement. It is vital to remember that folate and folic acid, its synthetic version, are not the same thing. Folate is a natural form of the vitamin, whereas folic acid is a synthetic variant that is routinely added to fortified meals and supplements.

One of the most significant advantages of folate in prenatal nutrition is its function in avoiding neural tube abnormalities. Neural tube abnormalities are birth anomalies that disrupt the development of the brain and spinal cord and may result in major health issues for the kid. Folate is required for the normal closure of the neural tube during the early stages of fetal development, and a shortage of folate in the mother's diet may raise the chance of neural tube defects.

In addition to avoiding neural tube anomalies, folate also plays a key role in the production of red blood cells and the prevention of anemia. Anemia is a frequent complication in pregnancy that happens when the body does not have enough red blood cells to transport oxygen to the body's tissues. Folate helps to form red blood cells, which is vital for sustaining a healthy pregnancy and avoiding anemia.

Furthermore, folate also helps to maintain the mother's immune system and minimize the risk of pre-eclampsia. Pre-eclampsia is a dangerous illness that may arise in pregnancy and is characterized by high blood pressure, edema, and protein in the urine. Folate serves to boost the immune system and prevent inflammation, which may minimize the risk of pre-eclampsia.

It is crucial to highlight that many women do not eat enough folate in their diet, which might raise the risk of birth abnormalities and other health issues. To ensure that pregnant women eat a suitable quantity of folate, it is suggested that they start taking a prenatal vitamin supplement that includes folate many months before becoming pregnant. In addition, it is also suggested that women continue to take a folate supplement during pregnancy to ensure that their developing baby receives the nutrients it requires for normal growth.

In conclusion, folate is an essential vitamin for proper prenatal nutrition. It is involved in various essential processes in the body and provides significant advantages for both the mother and the developing baby. By ingesting an adequate quantity of folate, pregnant women may guarantee that their developing baby obtains the nutrients it needs for healthy development and lower the chance of birth defects and other health issues. So, it is advised for pregnant women to have a balanced diet that is high in folate-rich foods, such as leafy green vegetables, legumes, nuts, and fruits, and to take a prenatal vitamin supplement that includes folate.

B. Iron

Iron is an important micronutrient that is crucial for good prenatal nutrition. During pregnancy, a woman's iron needs rise dramatically to support the growth and development of the baby, placenta, and maternal tissues. Adequate iron consumption helps to avoid maternal anemia, which may have detrimental implications for mother and fetal health.

Iron is a vital component of hemoglobin, a protein present in red blood cells that delivers oxygen from the lungs to the tissues. During pregnancy, the amount of blood in a woman's body rises to support the development of the baby, which leads to an increased requirement for iron. The placenta also needs iron to generate placental heme, which is crucial for the transport of oxygen and nutrients from the mother to the baby.

Maternal anemia is a frequent condition during pregnancy and may arise when a woman does not ingest enough iron to fulfill her increasing demands. Symptoms of anemia include exhaustion, weakness, and shortness of breath, which may significantly impair a woman's quality of life and capacity to conduct everyday tasks. In extreme situations, anemia during pregnancy may lead to early delivery, low birth weight, and other issues.

To maintain normal prenatal nutrition, it is necessary for pregnant women to eat enough levels of iron from a range of sources. Good dietary sources of iron include red meat, chicken, fish, beans, lentils, tofu, fortified cereals, and dark leafy greens. Iron from animal sources is more readily absorbed by the body compared to plant-based sources, hence it is suggested that pregnant women take at least two meals of animal-based iron sources each week.

In addition to food sources, pregnant women may also benefit from taking an iron supplement, which may assist to fulfill their increased iron needs. Supplements should be used under the guidance of a healthcare expert, since taking too much iron may be dangerous. It is also crucial to remember that iron absorption may be impeded by certain meals and drinks, such as tea, coffee, and calcium-rich foods. To increase iron absorption, it is advisable to take iron supplements on an empty stomach or with a source of vitamin C, such as orange juice.

Pregnant women should also take efforts to decrease the risk of iron loss, since this may also contribute to maternal anemia. Blood loss after birth and menstruation are the two primary causes of iron loss during pregnancy. To limit blood loss during delivery, women might consider adopting active management of the third stage of labor, which includes the use of uterotonic medications and controlled cord traction to prevent blood loss. To limit monthly blood loss, women should utilize a dependable type of birth control to avoid unplanned pregnancy.

In conclusion, iron is an essential micronutrient for healthy prenatal nutrition, as it promotes the growth and development of the baby and helps to avoid maternal anemia. Pregnant women should eat enough levels of iron from a range of sources and consider taking an iron supplement under the guidance of a healthcare expert. To increase iron absorption and limit iron loss, women should also take efforts to prevent blood loss during birth and menstruation. By following these suggestions, pregnant women may help to ensure that they and their growing baby get the iron they need for good health and well-being.

C. Calcium

Calcium is a critical vitamin that plays a significant role in prenatal nutrition, and its value cannot be emphasized. Calcium is important for the construction and maintenance of healthy bones and teeth in both the mother and the growing baby. A lack of calcium during pregnancy may lead to serious health concerns, including an increased risk of osteoporosis later in life, pre-eclampsia, and low birth weight in the infant.

In pregnancy, the body's requirement for calcium rises while the fetus is growing and forming bones. A pregnant woman's daily calcium needs doubles from 1000mg to 1300mg, which is the equivalent of three to four servings of calcium-rich meals. Adequate calcium consumption during pregnancy is needed for the appropriate construction of the baby's skeleton and to maintain the mother's increased blood volume.

Dairy products are the finest providers of calcium, and pregnant women should strive to consume at least three servings of dairy every day. Milk, yogurt, and cheese are all good sources of calcium, and may be readily integrated into a well-balanced diet. Other calcium-rich foods include almonds, leafy greens, sardines, and tofu.

For women who are lactose intolerant or follow a vegan diet, alternate forms of calcium may be provided via fortified dairy alternatives, such as soy milk and tofu, and calcium-enriched orange juice. Additionally, calcium supplements may be taken in the form of tablets or gummies, but it is vital to contact a healthcare expert before beginning any supplement plan.

In addition to its involvement in bone production, calcium is also important for the normal functioning of muscles and nerves, and it plays a key role in blood clotting and control of the heart's rhythm. During pregnancy, calcium helps to control the mother's blood pressure, which is necessary for the health and well-being of both the mother and the baby.

Despite its significance, calcium shortages are frequent in pregnancy, especially in women who have low dietary calcium intake or those who suffer from malabsorption problems. Women who have a family history of osteoporosis or who smoke or drink large quantities of coffee or alcohol are also at increased risk of having calcium shortages.

In conclusion, calcium is a key vitamin that plays a significant role in prenatal nutrition, and its significance cannot be emphasized. Pregnant women should attempt to take at least three servings of calcium-rich foods or calcium-enriched dairy alternatives each day, in addition to a well-balanced diet, to ensure that they and their growing fetus get enough quantities of this critical vitamin. Consultation with a healthcare expert is always important, especially for individuals contemplating calcium supplements, to ensure that their unique requirements are addressed.

D. Vitamin D

Vitamin D is one of the necessary micronutrients that play a key role in maintaining optimum health and wellbeing, particularly during pregnancy. As a fat-soluble vitamin, vitamin D is vital in regulating the body's absorption and metabolism of calcium, which is necessary for the formation and maintenance of healthy bones.

During pregnancy, appropriate consumption of vitamin D is necessary for the correct growth and development of the baby, including the production of bones, teeth, and muscles. Moreover, vitamin D also plays a key function in regulating the immune system, decreasing inflammation, and promoting general prenatal health.

The body may manufacture vitamin D via exposure to sunshine, but, this method of acquiring vitamin D is not always dependable, particularly for women who live in locations with low sun exposure or who have dark skin, since melanin limits the skin's capacity to make vitamin D. Moreover, many foods, such as dairy products, fatty fish, and egg yolks, are fortified with vitamin D, giving an extra supply of the vitamin.

It is suggested that pregnant women ingest 600-800 international units (IU) of vitamin D per day, which may be gained from food sources or supplementation. Women who are pregnant or nursing should contact their healthcare physician before commencing any supplements plan.

Adequate vitamin D consumption during pregnancy has been connected with various health advantages, including:

Improved prenatal growth and development: Vitamin D aids in the appropriate construction of bones and teeth, as well as the control of muscle growth in the fetus.

Reduced risk of gestational diabetes: Vitamin D has been found to have a protective impact against the development of gestational diabetes, a disease that affects pregnant women and may have major consequences for both the mother and the baby.

Improved immunological function: Vitamin D has a critical role in regulating the immune system, which is particularly essential during pregnancy when the body is more vulnerable to infections.

Reduced risk of pre-eclampsia: Pre-eclampsia is a dangerous condition that may arise during pregnancy and can have catastrophic repercussions for both the mother and the baby. Adequate vitamin D consumption has been connected with a lower incidence of preeclampsia.

Improved cardiovascular health: Vitamin D has been found to have a preventive impact against cardiovascular disease, which is particularly significant during pregnancy when circulatory changes occur.

In conclusion, vitamin D is an important micronutrient that plays a key role in maintaining optimum health and welfare throughout pregnancy. Adequate consumption of vitamin D may aid promote fetal growth and development, lower the risk of gestational diabetes, increase immunological function, minimize the risk of pre-eclampsia, and improve cardiovascular health. Pregnant women should aim to receive enough vitamin D via food sources or supplementation, under the advice of a healthcare provider.

Chapter 3: Eating for Two: Meal Planning and Portion Control

A. Adequate Caloric Intake

Adequate calorie intake is a vital part of meal planning and portion management for good prenatal nutrition. The recommended daily caloric intake for pregnant women is normally approximately 2,400 to 2,800 calories, depending on the women's beginning weight, age, and amount of physical activity. This increased caloric need is important to support the growth and development of the fetus, as well as to maintain the health and energy levels of the mother.

Portion management is similarly vital, as overeating or undereating may severely affect both the mother and the fetus. Consuming too many calories may lead to excessive weight gain, which can raise the risk of gestational diabetes, hypertension, and other issues. On the other side, ingesting too few calories may result in malnutrition, which can affect both the mother and the baby, and raise the chance of birth abnormalities.

When preparing meals, it is vital to pick nutrient-dense foods that supply the required vitamins, minerals, and essential fatty acids needed for good prenatal nutrition. Foods that are rich in protein, iron, calcium, and folic acid are very vital. Some examples of these sorts of foods are lean meats, poultry, fish, dairy products, legumes, whole grains, and leafy greens.

Protein is extremely vital for pregnant women, since it is required for the development and repair of tissues, and for the creation of hormones, enzymes, and antibodies. Lean meats, poultry, fish, eggs, dairy products, and legumes are all rich sources of protein. It is crucial to incorporate a variety of these foods in your diet to ensure that you are obtaining a comprehensive spectrum of necessary amino acids.

Iron is also a critical vitamin for pregnant women, since it is required to form hemoglobin, which delivers oxygen to the baby. Good sources of iron include lean meats, chicken, fish, beans, lentils, tofu, and fortified cereals. To enhance iron absorption, it is necessary to consume iron-rich meals in conjunction with foods that are high in vitamin C, such as citrus fruits, tomatoes, and bell peppers.

Calcium is another crucial vitamin for pregnant women, since it is required for the development of the fetus's bones and teeth, as well as for the mother's own bones. Good sources of calcium include dairy products, such as milk, cheese, and yogurt, as well as leafy greens, such as spinach and kale.

Folic acid is another crucial vitamin for pregnant women, since it is required for the development of the fetus's neurological system. Good sources of folic acid include leafy greens, such as spinach and kale, as well as fortified cereals, breads, and pasta. It is also suggested that women take a daily prenatal vitamin that includes folic acid.

In addition to selecting nutrient-dense meals, it is crucial to pay attention to portion sizes. Eating too much of any one meal may lead to excessive weight gain and raise the risk of gestational diabetes and hypertension. An excellent strategy to manage portion sizes is to use smaller plates and bowls, and to eat slowly and deliberately, paying attention to your hunger and fullness signals.

Finally, it is crucial to keep hydrated throughout pregnancy, since dehydration may affect both the mother and the child. Aim to drink at least 8 glasses of water a day, and to minimize your consumption of sugary beverages, such as soda and fruit juice. Instead, choose for water, unsweetened tea, or low-fat milk.

In conclusion, sufficient calorie intake and portion management are critical parts of meal planning for good prenatal nutrition. By selecting nutrient-dense meals, paying attention to portion sizes, and keeping hydrated, pregnant women may guarantee that they are given.

B. Food Groups to Focus On

Prenatal diet is vital for the health and development of both the mother and the baby. Proper meal planning and portion management may help ensure that pregnant moms are obtaining the required nutrients for a healthy pregnancy. Here are several dietary categories that should be a priority for optimum prenatal nutrition:

Fruits and Vegetables: Fruits and vegetables are key sources of vitamins, minerals, and fiber. Expectant moms should strive for at least five servings of fruits and vegetables every day. Some of the greatest selections are leafy greens, berries, citrus fruits, and colorful veggies like carrots, sweet potatoes, and bell peppers.

Whole Grains: Whole grains are rich in fiber and vital minerals including iron, folic acid, and B-vitamins. Expectant moms should choose whole-grain bread, rice, pasta, and cereal. Whole grain products are also a fantastic source of energy, which may help overcome weariness during pregnancy.

Lean Proteins: Lean proteins, such as chicken, fish, tofu, and beans, are necessary for the growth and development of the infant. Expectant moms should strive for at least two meals of lean protein every day. Fish, in particular, is an excellent source of omega-3 fatty acids, which are crucial for brain and eye development.

Dairy Products: Dairy products, including milk, cheese, and yogurt, are high in calcium and other key elements like vitamin D, which are required for healthy bones. Expectant moms should strive for at least three servings of dairy every day.

Healthy Fats: Healthy fats, including those found in nuts, seeds, and avocados, are vital for the baby's brain development and general health. Expectant moms should strive for at least two servings of healthy fats every day. It is also crucial to pay attention to portion management during pregnancy. Expectant moms should strive to eat smaller, more frequent meals throughout the day to help maintain their energy levels stable and prevent overeating. They should also avoid missing meals, since this may contribute to overeating and weight gain.

In addition to concentrating on these dietary categories, pregnant moms should also avoid specific foods that might be detrimental during pregnancy. These include raw or undercooked foods, seafood with high amounts of mercury, and some varieties of cheese that may carry hazardous germs. Caffeine should also be restricted to 200 mg per day, since high caffeine consumption has been associated with an increased risk of miscarriage and low birth weight.

In conclusion, careful meal planning and quantity management are critical for healthy pregnancy nutrition. Expectant moms should concentrate on eating a range of nutrient-rich meals from the five food categories outlined above, while also avoiding specific items that may be hazardous. With the correct diet, pregnant moms may promote their own health and the health and development of their infant

C. Managing Cravings and Aversions

Managing cravings and aversions is a crucial element of meal planning and quantity management for optimum prenatal nutrition. Pregnancy is a period of fast change for a woman's body and her dietary demands. To ensure that the baby grows appropriately, it is crucial that the mother consume a balanced diet that offers all the required vitamins, minerals, and nutrients. However, many women have desires and aversions during pregnancy, which may make eating a well-balanced diet difficult.

Cravings are overwhelming cravings to consume certain meals, whereas aversions are an avoidance of certain foods. These desires and aversions might be triggered by hormonal changes, emotional changes, or a mix of both. It's crucial to understand that although cravings and aversions are common throughout pregnancy, they are not a reliable sign of what the body needs nutritionally. For example, a woman may want ice cream and pickles, but this does not suggest that she needs more calcium or potassium in her diet.

The key to regulating cravings and aversions is to pick healthy meals that satisfy the body's demands. Rather than indulging in unhealthy or sugary meals, it's important to choose healthier options that still fulfill the appetite. For example, if a lady is seeking something sweet, she may consider eating fresh fruit or a tiny portion of dark chocolate. If she's seeking something crunchy, she may try eating raw veggies or air-popped popcorn.

In terms of portion management, it's recommended to consume modest, regular meals throughout the day rather than big, heavy meals. This helps to manage blood sugar levels, avoid overeating, and lessen the risk of heartburn, indigestion, and other digestive difficulties that are prevalent during pregnancy. Additionally, it's crucial to drink enough water throughout the day to help keep the body hydrated and minimize cravings.

When it comes to meal planning, it's crucial to concentrate on consuming a range of nutrient-dense meals. A balanced diet should contain lots of fruits, vegetables, entire grains, lean meats, and healthy fats. Some of the greatest nutrient-dense foods during pregnancy include:

Fruits: Apples, bananas, oranges, berries, and pomegranates are all abundant in vitamins, minerals, and antioxidants.

Vegetables: Leafy greens, bell peppers, carrots, and sweet potatoes are all rich in vitamins and minerals.

Whole grains: Whole-grain breads, pasta, and brown rice are healthy sources of fiber and complex carbs.

Lean proteins: Chicken, fish, tofu, and lentils are rich sources of protein and assist to build and repair muscle.

Healthy fats: Avocados, nuts, seeds, and olive oil are fantastic sources of healthy fats that assist to keep the body feeling full and pleased.

It's also vital to restrict some meals during pregnancy, such as coffee, alcohol, and artificial sweeteners. Caffeine may induce increased heart rate, headaches, and difficulties sleeping. Alcohol may damage the growing infant, while artificial sweeteners can interfere with the body's capacity to control blood sugar levels.

In conclusion, regulating cravings and aversions is a critical element of meal planning and quantity management for optimum prenatal nutrition. By selecting nutritious foods, eating small, frequent meals, and concentrating on a balanced diet, women may ensure that they and their baby obtain all the required vitamins, minerals, and nutrients for a healthy pregnancy.

Chapter 4: Common Concerns and Challenges

A. Nausea and Morning Sickness

Pregnancy is a wonderful and exciting time, but it may also come with different problems, one of which being nausea and morning sickness. Nausea and morning sickness are highly prevalent during pregnancy, affecting roughly 50-90% of pregnant women. The symptoms may vary from moderate to severe and can have a substantial influence on a woman's everyday life and ability to maintain appropriate nutrition throughout pregnancy.

Nausea and morning sickness are hypothesized to be induced by hormonal changes in the body, notably the rise in human chorionic gonadotropin (hCG) and the hormone estrogen. The specific processes underlying this link are not fully known, however it is thought that the hormones may impact the digestive system and induce sensitivity to particular meals or scents.

It is vital for women who feel nausea and morning sickness to seek medical assistance and engage with a healthcare practitioner to identify strategies to control their symptoms. There are various techniques that might be useful, including:

Eating several, little meals throughout the day instead of three big ones

Avoiding rich, spicy, or acidic meals that may provoke symptoms

Snacking on bland, high-protein items such as crackers or toast

Drinking lots of water to keep hydrated

Avoiding triggers such as strong scents or particular meals

Taking prenatal vitamins before night or with a light snack to reduce nausea

Practicing relaxation methods such as deep breathing or meditation

In addition to these tactics, there are also various natural therapies that may assist ease discomfort. Some women find comfort from drinking ginger tea or taking ginger tablets, while others find relief by acupressure bracelets or aromatherapy. It is vital to contact a healthcare practitioner before attempting any new treatments, since some may interfere with existing drugs or be prohibited during pregnancy.

While nausea and morning sickness may be tough to cope with, it is essential to realize that they are a normal component of pregnancy and that most women suffer some degree of symptoms. Women who have extreme nausea and vomiting, known as hyperemesis gravidarum, may require medical therapy to help control their symptoms and maintain appropriate nutrition throughout pregnancy.

Optimal nutrition throughout pregnancy is vital for the health and well-being of both the mother and the growing child. It is advised that women maintain a balanced diet that contains a range of whole grains, fruits and vegetables, lean proteins, and healthy fats. Women should also make sure they are receiving enough of certain critical nutrients, including folic acid, iron, calcium, and omega-3 fatty acids.

Women who are suffering nausea and morning sickness may struggle to satisfy their nutritional requirements, particularly if they are having difficulties eating or keeping food down. It is crucial for these women to seek medical assistance and engage with a healthcare practitioner to identify strategies to manage their symptoms and maintain adequate nutrition. In certain situations, women may need to take a prenatal vitamin or other supplements to ensure they are receiving all the nutrients they need throughout pregnancy.

In conclusion, nausea and morning sickness are normal problems for many women during pregnancy. While these symptoms may be tough to manage, there are numerous tactics and natural therapies that can be useful in decreasing their effect. Women who have severe symptoms should seek medical assistance and work with a healthcare practitioner to ensure they are maintaining adequate nutrition throughout pregnancy. With the correct help and services, women may effectively manage their symptoms and experience a healthy pregnancy

B. Food Aversions and Cravings

Prenatal nutrition is a crucial part of a healthy pregnancy and has a substantial influence on the growth and development of the baby. As the baby depends on the mother's diet for important nutrients, it is necessary for pregnant moms to make sure that they are eating properly to assist the developing infant. However, food aversions and desires may offer a difficulty for many women when it comes to keeping a well-rounded and balanced diet during pregnancy. In this post, we will cover food aversions and cravings as a typical worry for healthy prenatal nutrition and how to handle them.

Food Aversions

Food aversions are a frequent experience for many expecting moms, and they often entail a strong disgust or aversion to particular meals. This may be related to hormonal changes that modify the taste buds and change the way that food tastes and smells. Aversions may occur to a broad variety of foods, including those that are typically considered healthy, such as vegetables and fruits, or those that are bad, such as junk food.

The advent of food aversions may lead a woman to lose her appetite and be unable to eat enough to satisfy her nutritional requirements. This may be a concern, particularly when the foods that are being avoided are rich in critical elements such as calcium, iron, and folic acid. This may result in vitamin deficits that can be hazardous to both the mother and the baby.

Food Cravings

Food cravings are another frequent emotion for expecting moms, and they entail a strong desire for a specific food or food type. Some women may desire sweet meals, such as sweets and ice cream, while others may prefer salty or spicy foods. Food cravings may be severe and can come at any moment of the day or night. Food cravings may also be an issue for prenatal nutrition as they may lead to an imbalanced diet and an overconsumption of harmful foods. For example, if a woman is continually seeking sweets, she may eat more sugar than she needs, which may result in weight gain and an increased risk of gestational diabetes.

Managing Food Aversions and Cravings

The first step in treating food aversions and cravings is to determine the underlying reason. Hormonal shifts are generally the major cause for both food aversions and cravings, therefore it is crucial to engage with a healthcare expert to manage these changes. They may also give recommendations on how to address dietary demands throughout pregnancy.

If food aversions are impacting the capacity to eat sufficiently, it may be useful to locate other sources of the nutrients that are being avoided. For example, if vegetables are being avoided, there are many other foods that contain essential vitamins and minerals, such as leafy greens, nuts, and legumes.

It is also crucial to listen to the body and eat when hungry. If a woman is feeling queasy or is having problems eating, it may be useful to consume small, frequent meals throughout the day. This may assist to enhance the total intake of critical nutrients and promote the development of the fetus.

When it comes to food cravings, it is essential to practice moderation. If a woman is desiring sweet or salty meals, it may be useful to pick healthier choices, such as fresh fruit or air-popped popcorn. It may also be helpful to limit the portion sizes of the cravings to reduce the overall calorie intake and prevent weight gain.

Food aversions and desires are significant concerns for pregnant moms when it comes to good prenatal nutrition. While these changes might be tough, there are various methods to handle them, including listening to the body, eating small, frequent meals, and seeking alternate sources of critical nutrients. With the help of a healthcare

C. Gestational Diabetes

Gestational diabetes is a kind of diabetes that affects women during pregnancy. It happens when the body cannot manufacture enough insulin to satisfy the increasing needs of pregnancy. Insulin is a hormone that controls blood sugar levels. If insulin levels are low, blood sugar levels will increase, which may lead to gestational diabetes. The disease may create a number of health concerns for both the mother and baby, making it a frequent worry and obstacle for optimum prenatal nutrition.

Gestational diabetes affects up to 10% of all pregnancies, and the chance of acquiring the illness rises with age, obesity, and a family history of diabetes. Women with gestational diabetes are more prone to suffer difficulties during pregnancy, such as pre-eclampsia, big birth weight, and premature delivery. They are also more prone to acquire type 2 diabetes later in life.

The first step in controlling gestational diabetes is to regulate blood sugar levels with a nutritious diet and physical exercise. A balanced diet should contain whole grains, fruits and vegetables, lean meats, and healthy fats. Women with gestational diabetes should attempt to consume modest, frequent meals throughout the day to keep blood sugar levels steady.

Physical exercise is also crucial for regulating blood sugar levels. Regular exercise, such as a 30-minute walk each day, may help manage insulin levels and enhance overall health. Women with gestational diabetes should also test their blood sugar levels often to ensure that they are within a safe range.

In addition to nutrition and exercise, women with gestational diabetes may also need to take insulin injections to maintain blood sugar levels. Insulin treatment may help manage blood sugar levels, but it is vital to follow a healthcare professional's recommendations carefully to prevent low blood sugar levels.

Prenatal vitamins and minerals are particularly crucial for good prenatal nutrition, especially for women with gestational diabetes. Folic acid, iron, and calcium are needed for the growth of the fetus, and these nutrients should be taken in addition to a balanced diet. Women with gestational diabetes should also watch their weight increase throughout pregnancy, since excessive weight gain may lead to problems and difficulty with insulin administration.

Gestational diabetes might potentially impair the birth of the baby. Women with gestational diabetes are more likely to need induction of labor, cesarean birth, or a lengthier hospital stay following delivery. They are also more likely to experience difficulties after birth, such as postpartum depression, and are at a greater risk of acquiring type 2 diabetes later in life.

In conclusion, gestational diabetes is a frequent issue and obstacle for appropriate prenatal nutrition, since it may create a number of health concerns for both the mother and baby. Women with gestational diabetes should regulate blood sugar levels with a nutritious diet, physical exercise, and insulin treatment if required. They should also check their weight growth and take prenatal vitamins and minerals to help the development of the baby. With correct treatment, women with gestational diabetes may have a successful pregnancy and delivery, and lower the risk of long-term health concerns for themselves and their baby.

D. Overweight or Underweight Concerns

Pregnancy is a key phase in a woman's life, when the appropriate diet is important to guarantee the health and wellness of the mother and her unborn child. The mother's body goes through many physical, emotional, and hormonal changes throughout pregnancy, making it necessary to maintain a balanced and healthy diet. Overweight or underweight issues are one of the main difficulties experienced by pregnant women, and they may greatly impair prenatal nutrition and health.

Overweight Concerns

Overweight and obesity are becoming a significant issue among pregnant women, with the incidence of overweight and obese pregnant women increasing globally. Overweight and obesity in pregnancy may lead to various issues, including gestational diabetes, high blood pressure, preeclampsia, and birth of a big baby. Moreover, overweight and obesity in pregnancy might raise the chance of obesity and other health issues in the infant later in life.

The first trimester of pregnancy is a significant phase, since the creation of essential organs takes place during this time. Overweight and obese women have a greater risk of gestational diabetes, which may lead to high blood sugar levels in the mother and result in significant infant growth. A big baby raises the chance of problems during delivery and increases the risk of complications for both the mother and the infant.

During the second trimester, the mother's body undergoes significant changes, and it becomes increasingly difficult to maintain a good diet and exercise program. Overweight and obese women are at increased risk of gestational hypertension, which may progress to pre-eclampsia, a disease marked by high blood pressure and protein in the urine. Preeclampsia may be harmful for both the mother and the baby, leading to early birth and other issues.

In the third trimester, overweight and obese women are at increased risk of having a big baby, which may increase the risk of difficulties during delivery, including cesarean section, extended labor, and birth damage.

Underweight Concerns

Underweight women also face considerable hazards during pregnancy, including an increased chance of early delivery, low birth weight, and a greater risk of pregnancy problems. Low birth weight is a serious public health problem since it is related with higher morbidity and death in newborns and children.

Underweight women are generally undernourished and have reduced amounts of critical vitamins and minerals, including iron, calcium, and folic acid. These vitamins and minerals are needed for the proper development of the baby and the mother, and their shortage may lead to numerous pregnancy problems.

In the first trimester, underweight women are at increased risk of suffering a miscarriage, since the body may not have enough nutrition to nourish the developing baby. Underweight women are also at increased risk of suffering anemia during pregnancy, since they have lower amounts of iron, which is required for healthy blood synthesis. Anemia may contribute to tiredness, weakness, and an increased risk of early birth.

During the second trimester, underweight women are at increased risk of having a low birth weight baby, since the infant may not acquire enough nutrients to sustain growth and development. Low birth weight newborns are at increased risk of health issues, including respiratory distress syndrome, hypoglycemia, and a higher chance of mortality.

In the third trimester, underweight women are at increased risk of suffering difficulties during delivery, including early delivery and low birth weight. Underweight women are also at increased risk of having a tiny baby, which may raise the risk of difficulties during delivery and result in a higher risk of health issues in the kid later in life.

Overweight and underweight issues are key problems for optimum prenatal nutrition and health. Both disorders might raise the risk of pregnancy problems.

Chapter 5: Supplements and Food Fortification

A. Folic Acid

Folic acid is a B-vitamin that is needed for the growth and development of an unborn infant. Prenatal nutrition is critical for a healthy pregnancy, and folic acid is one of the most important nutrients for good fetal growth. In this article, we will explore the relevance of folic acid in prenatal nutrition, how it may be gotten via food fortification and supplements, and why it is necessary for a healthy pregnancy.

Folic acid is an essential vitamin in the early stages of pregnancy, playing a fundamental function in the formation of the neural tube. The neural tube creates the baby's brain and spinal cord, and if it does not shut correctly, it may result in neural tube abnormalities

(NTDs) such as spina bifida. Folic acid may assist to avoid various NTDs by helping to create healthy neural tissue and lowering the risk of NTDs by up to 70%.

Folic acid may also assist to prevent various birth problems such as cleft lip and palate, heart issues, and limb defects. In addition, folic acid has been associated with increased cognitive performance in children and a decreased risk of preterm delivery and low birth weight.

Food fortification is one technique to guarantee that you are receiving enough folic acid in your diet during pregnancy. Folic acid is added to meals such as bread, pasta, rice, and cereal to assist improve the consumption of this crucial vitamin. Some nations, such as the United States, have required fortification schemes to guarantee that women of reproductive age are receiving adequate folic acid. In other countries, food fortification is optional, thus it is necessary to check the label of the food you are eating to determine whether it has been fortified with folic acid.

In addition to dietary fortification, folic acid supplements are also available. These supplements are created exclusively for pregnant women and may supply the required daily amount of folic acid in one easy dosage. Some prenatal vitamins also include folic acid, so if you are taking a prenatal vitamin, you are likely receiving enough folic acid.

It is suggested that women who are hoping to get pregnant take 400 micrograms of folic acid each day, commencing at least one month before conception. This dosage may be raised to 600 to 800 mcg per day during pregnancy. It is vital to contact a healthcare practitioner before taking any supplements to establish the proper quantity for your unique requirements.

While folic acid is a necessary component for a healthy pregnancy, it is crucial to note that it should not be taken in high doses. Taking too much folic acid might interfere with the absorption of other critical minerals, such as iron and vitamin B12. It is also crucial to remember that folic acid pills should not be used as a replacement for a balanced diet that includes a range of nutrient-rich foods.

In conclusion, folic acid is a critical component for proper prenatal nutrition and should be a part of every woman's pregnant diet. It may be received via food fortification or supplements, and it is necessary to contact a healthcare expert to establish the proper quantity for your unique requirements. By taking folic acid, women may assist to guarantee a healthy pregnancy and lower the chance of birth abnormalities and other pregnancy issues.

B. Iron Supplements

Iron supplements and food fortification play a critical role in supporting proper prenatal nutrition. Pregnant women need to eat enough levels of iron in their diet to support the growth and development of their fetus. However, many women fail to satisfy their iron levels via food alone and need extra supplementation.

Iron is a vital mineral needed by the body to form hemoglobin, which is responsible for delivering oxygen to cells and tissues. During pregnancy, the body's iron demands rise dramatically owing to the development of the baby and the placenta. An appropriate quantity of iron is important for the production of red blood cells in both the mother and the fetus. Low iron levels during pregnancy may lead to iron-deficiency anemia, which is connected with several health issues.

Food fortification is a technique of adding vital vitamins and minerals, especially iron, to basic food products. This kind of supplementing is helpful in increasing the nutritional status of populations and lowering the incidence of nutrient deficiencies. The most typically fortified food products are cereal, wheat, and pasta. By ingesting these fortified food products, pregnant women may satisfy their daily iron needs without depending entirely on dietary sources.

Iron supplements, on the other hand, offer a more direct technique to augment iron consumption. These supplements come in numerous formats, including pills, capsules, and liquid versions. Pregnant women are generally recommended iron supplements by their doctor or obstetrician. The suggested dosage of iron supplements varies based on the individual's demands and the degree of their anemia.

There are two kinds of iron supplements available on the market - heme iron and nonheme iron. Heme iron is generated from animal sources and is more readily absorbed by the body compared to non-heme iron. Non-heme iron, on the other hand, is produced from plant sources and is not as readily absorbed by the body. To increase the absorption of nonheme iron, it is advisable to eat it together with a source of vitamin C, such as orange juice.

It is crucial to highlight that iron supplementation is not without adverse effects. Common side effects include constipation, nausea, and upset stomach. To reduce these adverse effects, it is advisable to take iron supplements with a meal and to drink lots of water.

In conclusion, iron supplements and dietary fortification serve a critical role in maintaining proper prenatal nutrition. Pregnant women should maintain a balanced diet that includes iron-rich food products and, if required, augment their iron consumption with iron supplements. It is vital to contact a healthcare expert before commencing any supplementation program, since excessive iron consumption may potentially have harmful consequences on health. By maintaining appropriate iron intake throughout pregnancy, women may promote the growth and development of their child and prevent the difficulties associated with iron-deficiency anemia.

C. Vitamin

Vitamin supplementation and food fortification are crucial measures for maintaining appropriate prenatal nutrition. Pregnancy is a period of increased dietary need for both the mother and the developing baby. During this period, it is crucial for women to maintain a balanced diet that includes all the critical nutrients for optimum fetal growth and development. In rare circumstances, however, dietary sources alone may not match the increased nutritional needs, making vitamin supplementation and food fortification required.

Vitamin supplementation during pregnancy is necessary to fulfill the increased demand for particular vitamins and minerals that play a key role in fetal growth and development. Some of the most critical vitamins during pregnancy are folic acid, iron, and calcium.

Folic acid is vital for avoiding birth abnormalities of the baby's brain and spine. It is suggested that all women of reproductive age ingest at least 400 micrograms of folic acid daily, and raise this to 600 micrograms during pregnancy. Women who have a history of having infants with neural tube abnormalities are generally recommended to ingest even larger amounts of folic acid. Folic acid pills are commonly accessible, and many prenatal vitamins include the needed quantity.

Iron is necessary for the development of the fetus's blood cells and placenta. Iron-deficiency anemia is a frequent concern during pregnancy, and supplementation might help avoid this. Women are encouraged to take at least 27 mg of iron per day during pregnancy, and supplements are generally prescribed to satisfy this need.

Calcium is crucial for the development of the fetus's bones and teeth. Calcium supplements are typically prescribed for women who do not eat appropriate levels of calcium in their diet. During pregnancy, women are encouraged to ingest at least 1000 mg of calcium every day.

In addition to vitamin supplementation, food fortification is another key technique for maintaining good prenatal nutrition. Food fortification includes adding vitamins and minerals to regularly eaten foods, such as bread and cereal, to improve the nutritious value.

One of the most frequent instances of food fortification is the addition of folic acid to enhanced flour and other grain products. This fortification has proved beneficial in lowering the occurrence of neural tube abnormalities in various nations. Other foods that are typically fortified with folic acid include breakfast cereals, pasta, and rice.

Iron fortification is also routinely used in several countries to avoid iron-deficiency anemia. Foods such as fortified cereals, bread, and pasta are typically enhanced with iron to assist fulfill the increased need for iron during pregnancy.

Food fortification is a key technique for ensuring that women have access to vital nutrients, even if they do not eat a balanced diet. This is particularly crucial in nations where food sources alone may not offer appropriate levels of nutrients.

In conclusion, vitamin supplementation and dietary fortification are critical measures for maintaining good prenatal nutrition. These measures assist to fulfill the increased need for key nutrients during pregnancy, such as folic acid, iron, and calcium, and help to avoid birth abnormalities and other health difficulties. Women are recommended to talk to their healthcare professional about their unique nutritional requirements during pregnancy, and to follow a balanced diet and take necessary vitamin supplements as required.

D Fortification

Fortification is the process of adding micronutrients to food to boost its nutritional content. The purpose of fortification is to correct nutritional shortages in communities and promote public health. Prenatal nutrition is especially essential since the health and nutrition of the mother during pregnancy may have a substantial influence on the health and development of the baby. Food fortification may play a vital role in providing proper prenatal nutrition and avoiding nutritional deficits.

Micronutrient deficits are a prevalent concern among pregnant women, particularly in low-income nations. Iron and folate are two of the most frequent deficiencies, and both may have major effects for both the mother and the baby. Iron-deficiency anemia during pregnancy raises the risk of maternal morbidity and death, and may also contribute to low birth weight and developmental abnormalities in the child. Folate deficiency may raise the chance of neural tube malformations in the pregnancy, as well as other birth problems.

Food fortification is a cost-effective and scalable way to treat these inadequacies. Common foods that are fortified include wheat, rice, salt, and sugar. The nutrients supplied to these meals are selected based on the frequency of deficiencies in a specific population and the practicality of fortifying the diet. For example, wheat is often reinforced with iron and folic acid, whereas salt is fortified with iodine.

One crucial part of food fortification is ensuring that the nutrients are provided in proper proportions. Too little of a nutrient may not have a major influence, while too much might be harmful. It is also crucial to evaluate the bioavailability of the vitamin, since certain forms of a nutrient may not be efficiently absorbed by the body.

In addition to dietary fortification, prenatal vitamins may also play a role in healthy prenatal nutrition. Prenatal supplements often include a number of micronutrients, including iron, folic acid, and calcium, to promote the health of the mother and the baby. It is vital to contact a healthcare expert before beginning a prenatal supplement, since certain nutrients may be dangerous in big doses.

In conclusion, food fortification is a beneficial technique for boosting prenatal nutrition and reducing nutritional deficits. By adding key micronutrients to popular meals, fortification may help guarantee that pregnant women have access to the nutrition they need for a healthy pregnancy. Combined with a balanced diet and prenatal vitamins, food fortification may assist to ensure appropriate prenatal nutrition and support the health and development of the baby.

Conclusion

As we reach the conclusion of our trip studying the significance of optimum prenatal nutrition, it is essential to reflect on the myriad advantages and considerations involved in maintaining a successful pregnancy. The first and important part of prenatal nutrition is to concentrate on a well-balanced diet that is rich in nutrients, vitamins, and minerals that are needed for the growth and development of the baby. It is also vital to understand the function of specific foods and supplements that may assist in ensuring optimum health outcomes for both the mother and the fetus.

In terms of particular nutrients, the focus must be on ingesting adequate iron, folate, calcium, and omega-3 fatty acids, which are crucial in ensuring a healthy pregnancy. Additionally, it is vital to avoid some meals such as processed foods, artificial sweeteners, alcohol, and caffeine, which might have detrimental effects on the growing baby.

One crucial issue to consider in enhancing prenatal nutrition is the significance of personalized nutrition regimens. No two pregnancies are the same, and what may work for one woman may not work for another. As such, it is vital to contact a healthcare expert to identify the individual nutritional requirements for each woman and their pregnancy.

Moreover, it is vital to examine the influence of prenatal nutrition on future health outcomes. Research has shown that optimal nutrition during pregnancy may have long-lasting impacts on the health of both the mother and the child, lowering the risk of chronic disorders such as heart disease, diabetes, and obesity.

Additionally, adequate prenatal nutrition may also assist to lower the risk of issues during pregnancy, such as pre-eclampsia, gestational diabetes, and preterm delivery. This underscores the necessity of establishing a balanced diet before pregnancy and continuing during the gestational period.

In conclusion, proper prenatal nutrition is a vital part of maintaining a healthy pregnancy and supporting beneficial results for both the mother and the child. It is crucial to concentrate on a well-balanced diet, ingest needed nutrients, and avoid items that may have bad consequences. It is also vital to contact a healthcare physician to design tailored nutrition regimens, and to evaluate the long-term impact of prenatal nutrition on future health outcomes.

In light of all the aforementioned, we strongly suggest seeking out expert counsel from a registered dietitian or a healthcare practitioner to identify the appropriate nutrition plan for each pregnancy. By doing so, pregnant moms may secure the greatest potential health results for themselves and their developing baby.

In addition to obtaining expert counsel, we also encourage adding physical exercise into everyday routines, as this may benefit in boosting general health and wellness throughout pregnancy. Additionally, expecting moms should make an effort to manage stress and maintain a healthy lifestyle, which may favorably benefit the health of both the mother and the baby.

In conclusion, prenatal nutrition is a critical part of maintaining a healthy pregnancy and supporting excellent results for both the mother and the baby. By concentrating on a well-balanced diet, including physical exercise, and obtaining expert counseling, pregnant moms may take the essential measures towards supporting maximum health for themselves and their developing fetus

www.ingramcontent.com/pod-product-compliance
Lightning Source LLC
Chambersburg PA
CBHW061323250726

48653CB00039B/2365